YOGA
JOURNAL
BLUE

This book belongs to:

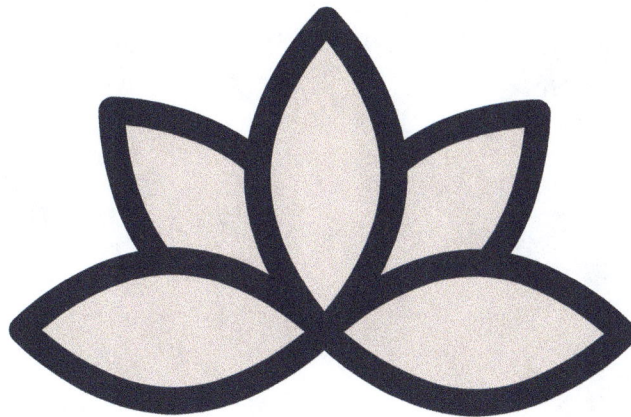

_____

GROUP / INDIVIDUAL

POSES PRACTICED

BODY & MIND PROGRESS

BEFORE

AFTER

CHAKRAS & AURA FIELDS

GROUP / INDIVIDUAL

POSES PRACTICED

BODY & MIND PROGRESS

BEFORE

AFTER

CHAKRAS & AURA FIELDS

GROUP / INDIVIDUAL

POSES PRACTICED ✓

BODY & MIND PROGRESS

BEFORE

AFTER

CHAKRAS & AURA FIELDS

GROUP / INDIVIDUAL

POSES PRACTICED ✓

BODY & MIND PROGRESS

BEFORE

AFTER

CHAKRAS & AURA FIELDS

POSES PRACTICED

BODY & MIND PROGRESS

BEFORE

AFTER

CHAKRAS & AURA FIELDS

GROUP / INDIVIDUAL

POSES PRACTICED ✓

BODY & MIND PROGRESS

BEFORE

AFTER

CHAKRAS & AURA FIELDS

POSES PRACTICED

BODY & MIND PROGRESS

BEFORE

AFTER

CHAKRAS & AURA FIELDS

GROUP / INDIVIDUAL

POSES PRACTICED ✓

BODY & MIND PROGRESS

BEFORE

AFTER

CHAKRAS & AURA FIELDS

GROUP / INDIVIDUAL

POSES PRACTICED

BODY & MIND PROGRESS

BEFORE

AFTER

CHAKRAS & AURA FIELDS

POSES PRACTICED

BODY & MIND PROGRESS

BEFORE

AFTER

CHAKRAS & AURA FIELDS

GROUP / INDIVIDUAL

POSES PRACTICED

BODY & MIND PROGRESS

BEFORE

AFTER

CHAKRAS & AURA FIELDS

GROUP / INDIVIDUAL

POSES PRACTICED

BODY & MIND PROGRESS

BEFORE

AFTER

CHAKRAS & AURA FIELDS

POSES PRACTICED

BODY & MIND PROGRESS

BEFORE

AFTER

CHAKRAS & AURA FIELDS

POSES PRACTICED

BODY & MIND PROGRESS

BEFORE

AFTER

CHAKRAS & AURA FIELDS

GROUP / INDIVIDUAL

POSES PRACTICED

BODY & MIND PROGRESS

BEFORE

AFTER

CHAKRAS & AURA FIELDS

POSES PRACTICED

BODY & MIND PROGRESS

BEFORE

AFTER

CHAKRAS & AURA FIELDS

POSES PRACTICED

BODY & MIND PROGRESS

BEFORE

AFTER

CHAKRAS & AURA FIELDS

POSES PRACTICED

BODY & MIND PROGRESS

BEFORE

AFTER

CHAKRAS & AURA FIELDS

POSES PRACTICED

BODY & MIND PROGRESS

BEFORE

AFTER

CHAKRAS & AURA FIELDS

POSES PRACTICED

BODY & MIND PROGRESS

BEFORE

AFTER

CHAKRAS & AURA FIELDS

GROUP / INDIVIDUAL

POSES PRACTICED

BODY & MIND PROGRESS

BEFORE

AFTER

CHAKRAS & AURA FIELDS

GROUP / INDIVIDUAL

POSES PRACTICED

BODY & MIND PROGRESS

BEFORE

AFTER

CHAKRAS & AURA FIELDS

GROUP / INDIVIDUAL

POSES PRACTICED

BODY & MIND PROGRESS

BEFORE

AFTER

CHAKRAS & AURA FIELDS

GROUP / INDIVIDUAL

POSES PRACTICED

BODY & MIND PROGRESS

BEFORE

AFTER

CHAKRAS & AURA FIELDS

POSES PRACTICED

BODY & MIND PROGRESS

BEFORE

AFTER

CHAKRAS & AURA FIELDS

GROUP / INDIVIDUAL

POSES PRACTICED

BODY & MIND PROGRESS

BEFORE

AFTER

CHAKRAS & AURA FIELDS

POSES PRACTICED

BODY & MIND PROGRESS

BEFORE

AFTER

CHAKRAS & AURA FIELDS

GROUP / INDIVIDUAL

POSES PRACTICED

BODY & MIND PROGRESS

BEFORE

AFTER

CHAKRAS & AURA FIELDS

GROUP / INDIVIDUAL

POSES PRACTICED

BODY & MIND PROGRESS

BEFORE

AFTER

CHAKRAS & AURA FIELDS

POSES PRACTICED

BODY & MIND PROGRESS

BEFORE

AFTER

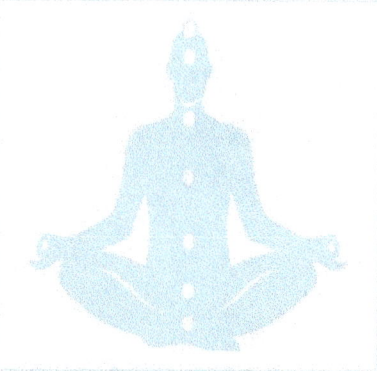

CHAKRAS & AURA FIELDS

GROUP / INDIVIDUAL

POSES PRACTICED

BODY & MIND PROGRESS

BEFORE

AFTER

CHAKRAS & AURA FIELDS

GROUP / INDIVIDUAL

POSES PRACTICED ✓

BODY & MIND PROGRESS

BEFORE

AFTER

CHAKRAS & AURA FIELDS

GROUP / INDIVIDUAL

POSES PRACTICED

BODY & MIND PROGRESS

BEFORE

AFTER

CHAKRAS & AURA FIELDS

GROUP / INDIVIDUAL

POSES PRACTICED ✓

BODY & MIND PROGRESS

BEFORE

AFTER

CHAKRAS & AURA FIELDS

POSES PRACTICED

BODY & MIND PROGRESS

BEFORE

AFTER

CHAKRAS & AURA FIELDS

GROUP / INDIVIDUAL

POSES PRACTICED

BODY & MIND PROGRESS

BEFORE

AFTER

CHAKRAS & AURA FIELDS

GROUP / INDIVIDUAL

POSES PRACTICED

BODY & MIND PROGRESS

BEFORE

AFTER

CHAKRAS & AURA FIELDS

POSES PRACTICED

BODY & MIND PROGRESS

BEFORE

AFTER

CHAKRAS & AURA FIELDS

GROUP / INDIVIDUAL

POSES PRACTICED

BODY & MIND PROGRESS

BEFORE

AFTER

CHAKRAS & AURA FIELDS

GROUP / INDIVIDUAL

POSES PRACTICED

BODY & MIND PROGRESS

BEFORE

AFTER

CHAKRAS & AURA FIELDS

POSES PRACTICED

BODY & MIND PROGRESS

BEFORE

AFTER

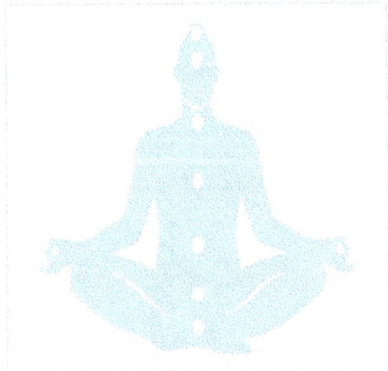

CHAKRAS & AURA FIELDS

POSES PRACTICED

BODY & MIND PROGRESS

BEFORE

AFTER

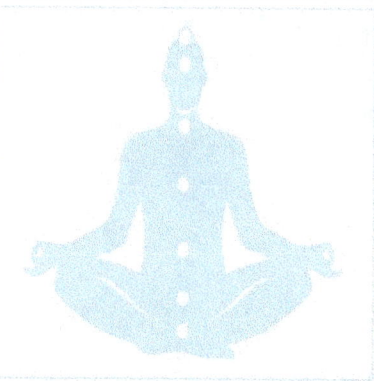

CHAKRAS & AURA FIELDS

POSES PRACTICED

BODY & MIND PROGRESS

BEFORE

AFTER

CHAKRAS & AURA FIELDS

GROUP / INDIVIDUAL

POSES PRACTICED ✓

BODY & MIND PROGRESS

BEFORE

AFTER

CHAKRAS & AURA FIELDS

GROUP / INDIVIDUAL

POSES PRACTICED

BODY & MIND PROGRESS

BEFORE

AFTER

CHAKRAS & AURA FIELDS

GROUP / INDIVIDUAL

POSES PRACTICED

BODY & MIND PROGRESS

BEFORE

AFTER

CHAKRAS & AURA FIELDS

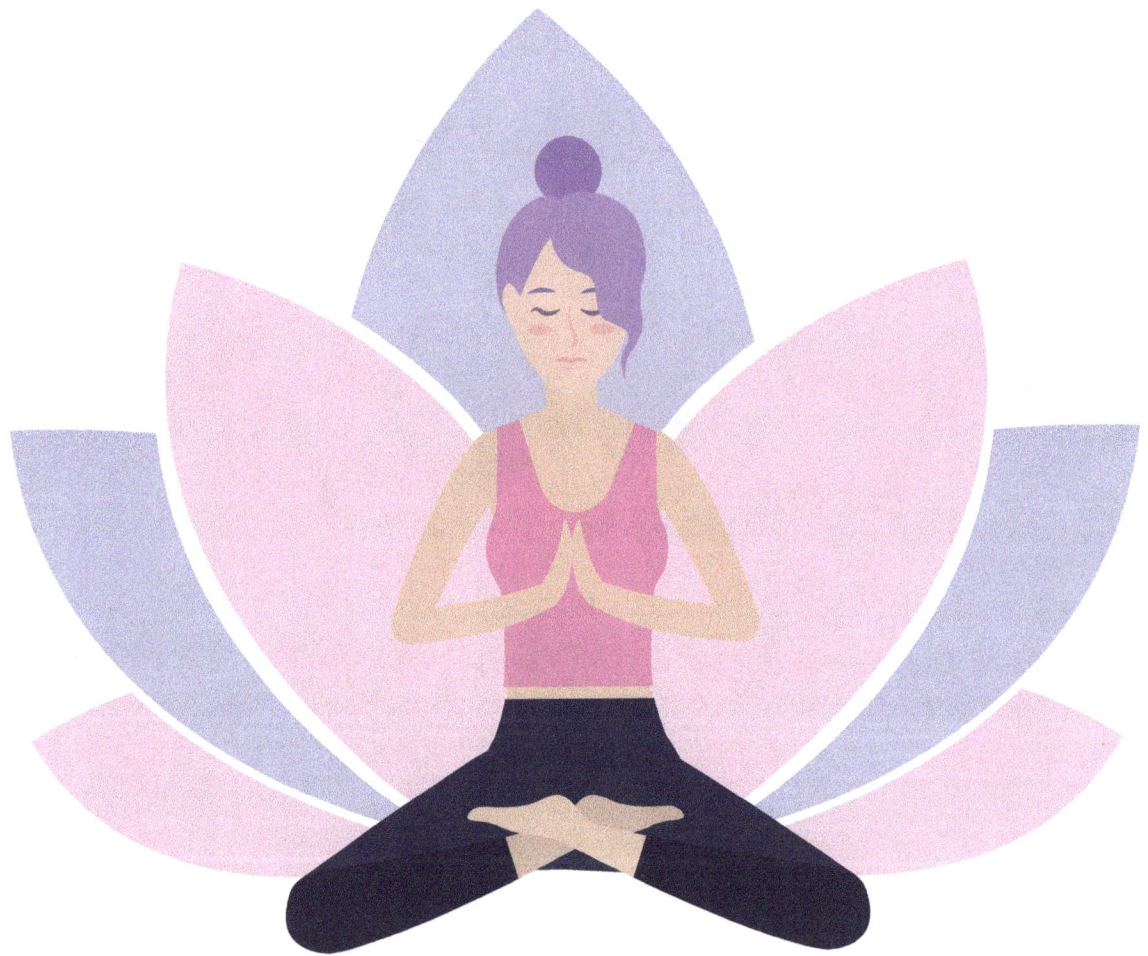

www.ingramcontent.com/pod-product-compliance
Lightning Source LLC
Chambersburg PA
CBHW080631030426

42336CB00018B/3152